Make Summer Go With A Bang

A Simple Guide To Barbecuing

Samantha Michaels

Table of Contents

Introduction

What methods we use for cooking will have an effect on the amount of nutrition the food provides us with. It doesn't matter if you spend money buying food with a low calorie content as soon as you choose to say deep fry the items not only will the amount of calories you consume be far greater, also you will find that they won't contain as many nutrients, minerals and vitamins your body needs in order to function at its optimum levels.

Furthermore any food deep-fried will not only be extremely fattening, but will contain high levels of cholesterol. Plus it will also contain other chemicals that can prove detrimental to your health and your body.

In recent years as the number of fast food restaurants offering deep fried food has increase so we find the incidents of obesity, diabetes and cardiovascular diseases has also increased. If you want to avoid weight problems or other health issues there are plenty of other healthy methods you can use for cooking your food such as grilling on a barbecue.

Most people of course tend to associate barbecuing with having fun, that involves a few alcoholic drinks as well as consuming some very fattening foods. However if you choose to barbecue your food you are actually eating food that is much healthier for you and which very few people realize. Today there are many physicians, dieticians as well as nutritionists who now recommend that barbecuing or grilling food is a much healthier way to cook food that it would be to deep fry them.

There are certain advantages to be gained from barbecuing more of your food.

The first is that when you barbecue food it will often contain far less fat that anything that has been immersed in oil even if you are using something like olive oil. Generally when cooking food on a barbecue it only requires a small amount of oil to be used to ensure that it doesn't stick to the grill. The amount you need to use is miniscule in comparison to what is required when it comes to frying it.

The second advantage to cooking on a barbecue is that if you want you can remove any fat from the meet before cooking commences. This will then help to reduce the amount of fat you are consuming which will help to ensure your cholesterol levels don't become too high.

The third advantage to be gained from barbecuing food is that it contains a much lower calorie content, compared to food that is cooked in the oven or on the hob. So perfect for those who are watching the calories because they are trying to lose weight.

The fourth advantage to cooking on a barbecue is that because you aren't using so much fat when cooking you are reducing the risk of developing certain illnesses or diseases. People who barbecue (grill) food are less likely to develop illnesses or diseases such as obesity, diabetes type 2, high blood pressure, heart disease or stroke.

Finally of course if you choose to grill food on a barbecue you are helping to ensure that more the vitamins, minerals and nutrients your body needs are retained in what you are eating. If you were to grill vegetables rather than boil or steam them you will find that they contain higher levels of vitamins and nutrients within them. The problem with boiling or steaming vegetables is that they drain a large number of the vitamins and nutrients out.

So as you can see above the reasons why eating barbecued food is such as healthy option. In this book we take a further look at what to do when it comes to purchasing a barbecue grill.

Chapter 1 - Pros & Cons Of Cooking On A Barbecue Grill

When it comes to cooking outdoors the most popular method is to use a barbecue grill. Quite a few of us do have experience of using such devices but generally will only cook on such when the weather is nice. So most of us tend to leave it outside to the elements and course end up having to buy a new one before summer commences because it has been neglected and left to rust.

In order for you to realize just how great using such equipment throughout the year can be we take a look at some of the pros and cons of cooking using a barbecue grill not just in the summer.

Pros of Cooking On a Barbecue Grill

1. You will find that cooking food on a barbecue grill tastes much more delicious. When you cook food on such a device the intense heat helps to caramelize the surface of it. As well as giving the food a much nicer color (a rich golden brown) you will also find it helps to bring out more of the raw foods wonderful flavors. Furthermore you can add other wonderful flavors to your food. For example using a wood smoker box with your gas or charcoal grill will help

to impart some lovely smoked wood flavor to the food.

2. You will often find that these types of devices are much more convenient to use. Not only are these types of devices readily available but also extremely easy to use. They do vary in price from basic models that cost only a few dollars to the more elaborate ones that come with a wide array of cool features that could cost you a couple of thousand dollars.

3. There are several kinds of barbecue grills now available. You can go for the more traditional charcoal models, which impart a different kind of flavor into your food. But of course setting them up can be quite messy, and you need to use the right sorts of equipment to help get the charcoal alight initially.

   Otherwise you can go for the more expensive models, which run off gas. As well as being a lot less messy to use they are also a lot easier to get up and running. You can if you want actually connect these devices to the mains gas line at your home so not only will they prove much cheaper to run, they will also prove to be much better for the environment especially if you home runs on natural gas. Plus of course you won't have to worry about buying replacement gas bottles.

   Also if you want to you could consider investing in one of the models that has infrared burners installed. As these have only recently come onto the market be aware that these are the most expensive to buy. But as they supply a very high intense heat when turned on they sear the food very quickly ensuring more of the juices are sealed inside. This in turn means that more of the nutrients, minerals and vitamins are being retained within the food as well.

4. When it comes to cooking on a barbecue you aren't limited to just putting meat or fish on it to grill. There are plenty of other cooking methods you can employ including direct heat or indirect heat cooking, along with smoking and rotisserie cooking. So this is a very versatile piece of equipment to use to create delicious tasting healthy meals for the whole family.

5. You will find that there are different styles of cooking that can be altered so that they can be cooked on a barbecue. As you will see at the end of this book there are numerous recipes, which you can use to create fantastic meals on a barbecue.

Cons of Cooking On a Barbecue Grill

There aren't that many cons of cooking on a barbecue grill. However below are some of the ones that a few people tend to complain about when barbecuing.

1. Of all the forms of cooking you can do these days this tends to be the messiest, especially if you are using a charcoal model. Also if you don't take care of your correctly after each

use, which means cleaning everything down then of course you are at risk of causing harm to others.

2. The problem with using a barbecue grill is that it takes time to get it up and running. Therefore if you want to prepare food in a matter of minutes then using a barbecue grill isn't going to be your best option. Of course that is only if you are using a charcoal fuelled model. If you are using a model that uses gas then of course it only takes a few minutes for the grill to reach the required temperature for you to then cook on it.

Chapter 2 - Types Of Barbecue Grills You Can Buy

If you have decided to replace your current barbecue grill with something new then you are going to find yourself spoilt for choice. In this chapter of this book we actually take a look at some of the kinds of barbecue grills now available.

Type 1 – Charcoal Barbecue Grill

This is of course the most common type of barbecue grill people consider purchasing as it tends to be the least expensive. Not only are these types of barbecue grills versatile but also the food cooked on them tastes absolutely wonderful. A charcoal model uses fuel that helps to produce long lasting heat so ensuring that every piece of food placed on it will be cooked to perfection.

However cooking on such models tends to be a lot messier and also will take a lot more time to prepare ready for use.

There are many different types of charcoal barbecue grills worth investing in. Below are some you may want to consider:

1. Weber Smokey Joe Grills (http://www.amazon.com/Weber-10020-Smokey-Silver-Charcoal/dp/B00004RALL/ref=sr_1_25?ie=UTF8&qid=1339405539&sr=8-25)
2. George Forman GGR50B Indoor/Outdoor Grill

(http://www.amazon.com/George-Foreman-GGR50B-Indoor-Outdoor/dp/B00004W499/ref=sr_1_2?ie=UTF8&qid=1339405381&sr=8-2)

3. Weber Performer Charcoal Grill (http://www.amazon.com/Weber-1421001-Performer-Charcoal-Grill/dp/B002M1PQZE/ref=sr_1_12?ie=UTF8&qid=1339405452&sr=8-12)

4. Grill Dome Large Charcoal Ceramic Grill Infinity Series (http://www.amazon.com/Grill-Dome-Charcoal-Ceramic-Infinity/dp/B005T072VQ/ref=sr_1_13?ie=UTF8&qid=1339405452&sr=8-13)

Type 2 – Gas Barbecue Grill

This type of barbecue tends to need a propane tank to be connected to it in order to provide the fuel. As well as these types of barbecues heating up a lot more quickly, they are much cleaner to use and also much easier to use. If you want to add a little more flavor to your food using a smoker box can prove extremely beneficial. As standard many now come fitted with a rotisserie attachment.

Below are some of the gas barbecue grills you may want to consider investing in.

1. Weber 586002 Q320 Portable Outdoor Propane Gas Grill (http://www.amazon.com/Weber-586002-Portable-Outdoor-

Propane/dp/B000WOVZ26/ref=sr_1_17?ie=
UTF8&qid=1339405814&sr=8-17)

2. Cajun Injector Propane Gas Pedestal Tower
   Grill   (http://www.amazon.com/Cajun-
   Injector-Propane-Pedestal-
   Tower/dp/B003V9CU8C/ref=sr_1_85?ie=UT
   F8&qid=1339405918&sr=8-85)

3. Char Broil Patio Bistro Infrared Gas Grill
   (http://www.amazon.com/Broil-Patio-Bistro-
   Infrared-
   Grill/dp/B002DM5DV4/ref=pd_sim_sbs_sg_
   1)

4. Jenn-AirÂ® Outdoor Gas Grill
   (http://www.amazon.com/Jenn-
   Air%C3%82%C2%AE-Outdoor-Gas-
   Grill/dp/B004WLCVQY/ref=sr_1_28?ie=UT
   F8&qid=1339406050&sr=8-28)

Type 3 – Natural Gas Barbecue Grill

This type of barbecue grill is able to plug directly into your homes natural gas line. So you don't need to worry about having to make sure that you have enough propane tanks to ensure that when using yours you don't run out of gas to cook with. Also this type of fuel burns much more cleanly so is far better for the environment than propane is. Today there are certain barbecue grills that have been made that can be specifically used with natural gas. However there are certain models that can also be converted over to using this form of fuel as well.

Below are some natural gas barbecue grills you may want to consider buying.

5. Weber 451101 Spirit E-210 Natural Gas Grill
(http://www.amazon.com/Weber-4511001-Spirit-E-210-Natural/dp/B001H1HOR8/ref=sr_1_10?ie=UTF8&qid=1339406279&sr=8-10)

6. Ducane 31732101 Affinity 3100 Natural Gas Grill
(http://www.amazon.com/Ducane-31732101-Affinity-Natural-Grill/dp/B001I8ZTZY/ref=sr_1_15?ie=UTF8&qid=1339406323&sr=8-15)

7. Minden Grill Company MMC1000 Master Natural Gas Grill
(http://www.amazon.com/Minden-Grill-Company-MMC1000-Natural/dp/B001NGO34Y/ref=sr_1_51?ie=UTF8&qid=1339406422&sr=8-51)

8. Broil King 987737 Sovereign 70 Natural Gas Grill
(http://www.amazon.com/987737-Sovereign-Natural-Rotisserie-Burner/dp/B004EBUTVG/ref=sr_1_84?ie=UTF8&qid=1339406496&sr=8-84)

Chapter 3 - Preparing Your Barbecue Grill For Cooking

When it comes to cooking food on a barbecue it is important that you prepare this equipment properly before you commence. Also you will find that when cooking on a barbecue grill it takes quite a bit of practice before you start to get things right.

In order to ensure that you cook food properly on a barbecue grill in this chapter of the book we look more closely at things you should be doing. Plus we also provide information about how to prepare either a charcoal or gas barbecue grill for cooking on.

The first things that need to be done when it comes to preparing your barbecue grill for cooking are as follows:

1. It is important that you make sure that your grill is clean before you even think about cooking on it. Nothing can be worse than placing a beautiful rib eye steak on yours to only find when eating it, that it tastes more like a piece of salmon.

   When it comes to cleaning your barbecue grill the best time to do it is when the grate is still hot after you have cooked on it. If you decide to wait until you choose to start cooking on yours there is the possibility of a flare up occurring as some of the scraps fall on to the heat below. Another thing you should do also to help reduce the amount of cleaning your barbecue needs after use is to spray or brush the grate with some vegetable oil. This will then help to prevent food from sticking to it especially when using marinades that contain ingredients such as honey in them.

2. The next thing you must do is to make sure that the grill is hot before you start cooking on it. Most people especially when using a gas barbecue grill will tend to start using it immediately. However it is far better if you allow it to heat up for around 15 to 30 minutes before you start using it. Doing this will help to ensure that the food will be cooked through properly.

3. You should spend time learning more about your barbecue grill, as each model is different, especially in relation to where the hot and cool spots are. If you know where these are then you can use them to your advantage when cooking on it.

Above we have offered you some basic tips about what needs to be done before you start cooking on your barbecue grill. Now let us take a look at what needs to be done to prepare a charcoal or gas barbecue grill for cooking on.

How To Prepare A Charcoal Barbecue Grill

You will need to make sure that you have the right tools for preparing your charcoal barbecue grill. Along with the barbecue grill you will also need a long match lighter or a butane barbecue lighter, a pair of tongs, some lighter fluid and good quality charcoal.

It is important to note that you should be using lump charcoal rather than briquettes. The problem with charcoal briquettes is that they contain certain chemicals to ensure that they burn at a constant rate. As a result some of these chemicals will transform into gas odors that then seep into the food being cooked on the grill and make it taste quite unpleasant.

Also you should consider using lump charcoal you will find cleaning your barbecue grill a lot easier as they don't leave so much mess because they don't leave as much ash behind. Also you will find that this type of charcoal has a much higher fire control rate as it is much more responsive to oxygen.

To prepare your charcoal grill for cooking on you need to carry out the following steps.

Step 1 – Create a cylinder using some newspaper. To help you make the right sort of cylinder you may find wrapping it around an empty bottle helps. Don't forget to take the bottle out before you place the cylinder of newspaper in to the center of the barbecue. Now very slowly place some of the charcoal around it and stack over it in a pyramid shape.

Step 2 – Once your pyramid of charcoal has been created douse it evenly with some of the barbecue lighter fluid. It is important that you read the instructions with the fluid fully and carefully. Also don't ever use gasoline or any other type of flammable liquid to get the charcoal burning.

If you would prefer not to use any type of lighter fluid to get your charcoal burning you may want to consider investing in a metal chimney starter. With this type of device you simply pile charcoal inside the cylinder and place it on top of the grid. Add some newspaper underneath it, which you then light.

Step 3 – After you have doused the charcoal in lighter fluid allow it time to soak in (around about a minute should do). Once this time has elapsed you can now light the charcoal with your long lighter match or the butane barbecue lighter you have purchased. As well as putting the flame towards the paper also put it close to the charcoal.

Step 4 – As soon as you can see that the paper and charcoal have ignited you need to let them burn for around 30 minutes. By this time they should start to be covered in a white ash.

Step 5 – As soon as you notice that there is white ash appearing on the charcoal you now need to spread it out evenly across the base of the barbecue. Once you have done this now the barbecue is now ready to start cooking on.

How To Prepare A Gas Barbecue Grill

The process of preparing your gas barbecue grill for cooking on starts immediately after it has been removed from the packaging it which it was developed and when it is being assembled. If you cure or season your gas barbecue grill before you start cooking on it you will find that it lasts a lot longer. You should be looking at spending at least an hour or two preparing the grill once removed from its packaging and has been assembled before you even consider using it for cooking.

Below are the steps you need to follow when not only preparing a new gas barbecue grill but also for when cooking on it.

Step 1 – After assembling your gas barbecue grill spend a little time wiping down all surfaces inside and out including the grate, grilling chamber and lid with a cloth or sponge that is soaked in hot water. After doing this allow the grill to dry out naturally.

Step 2 – The next thing you need to do is apply a very thin layer of vegetable oil or shortening to all surfaces. If you can place the oil in a bottle and spray it directly on to the surfaces of the barbecue grill. However if you are using shortening then apply it using a sheet of greaseproof paper.

Step 3 – Allow time for the oil or shortening to adhere to the surfaces of the barbecue grill. Then once this has happened you need to turn your gas barbecue on. Set the burners at a medium to low heat. Now close the lid and adjust the heat inside using the dials provided so that it remains at between 250 and 300 degrees Fahrenheit. Keep the lid closed for between 1 and 2 hours or until you notice that no smoke is being produced. When this occurs you should turn the heat off and leave the lid closed for a few minutes for things to cool down. Once it has cooled down and you open it up inside you will notice a dark protective coating has formed over the surfaces.

Only after this process has been completed will your gas barbecue grill be ready to use. Below we take you now through the steps required to prepare such equipment for cooking on.

Step 1 – If you haven't done previously whilst the gas barbecue grill is heating up remove grate and scrub vigorously to remove any debris or leftover food from when you used it previously. However it is far better if you actually clean the grate after each use, as it will help to prevent too much grease from building up on the grates surface. Also it will help to prevent debris from other meals cooked on your gas barbecue from adhering to the fresh food you have placed on it.

Step 2 – Once your grate is clean now you need to able a thin layer of vegetable oil to the surface of it. Make sure that you spray or brush the vegetable oil on to both sides of the grate. Then place it back inside the barbecue. Applying vegetable oil on to the grate each time it is used will help to leave some attractive grill marks on the surface of the food being cooked. If you can use a specially formulated vegetable oil spray for barbecues, as this is able to withstand much higher temperatures before it begins burning.

Step 3 – As soon as the grate is back in place now close the lid and let the grill heat up to a temperature of 350 degrees Fahrenheit. Once this temperature has been reached which should take around 15 minutes you can then start cooking on it.

Above we have shown you how to prepare both charcoal and gas barbecue grills for cooking on. However there are a couple of pieces of safety advice to remember as well when cooking on such equipment.

1. When cooking on a barbecue grill use fire resistant cooking gloves when handling the lid, vents or grates. This will then help to ensure that you won't get burnt seriously.
2. When it comes to handling any kind of food on your barbecue grill make sure that you use long handled tongs or a spatula. This will again help to prevent you getting injured when flare-ups occur.
3. To prevent any grease fires from happening make sure that you empty the barbecue's grease trap or tray on a regular basis, both during cooking and afterwards.

Chapter 4 - Tips For Preparing Food For The Barbecue

Most of us when the weather is good, especially in the summer like to spend as much time outdoors as possible. Certainly we also like to invite friends and family around to enjoy a barbecue with us. However it is important if you are going to invite people round that you make sure that you prepare all food to be served at such events properly. If you don't there is a risk of actually causing harm to others.

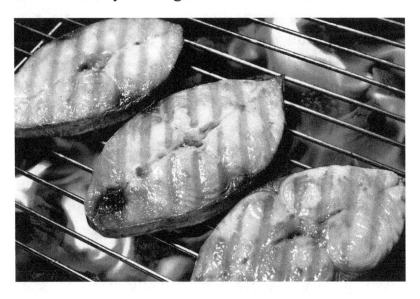

By following the tips offered below for preparing food for the barbecue not only can you avoid any disasters, but also ensure that everyone including you has a really great time.

Tip 1 – Make sure that you cook everything on your barbecue adequately. If you don't food that isn't cooked fully will retain certain times of bacteria that could make you and others ill. This is especially important when using food that has been thawed out after being frozen or is outside in the heat prior to it being cooked.

Tips 2 – To make sure that all food has been cooked through thoroughly invest in a good quality meat thermometer.

Tip 3 – When it comes to the handling of raw food make sure that you use separate utensils and plates. Also if you are handling any raw food make sure that you wash your hands before you say handle raw chicken and then raw fish. Plus after the food has been cooked make sure that you don't put it on to the plate on which raw food was held. As with your hands make sure that you wash all utensils and plates used for handling raw food before handling food that is cooked.

Tip 4 – Before you cook any vegetables, fish or poultry on your barbecue grill make sure that they have been thoroughly washed.

Tip 5 – Always leave raw food in the refrigerator (covered over) before you actually need to start cooking it. If you take it out before it is needed the heat outside will help even more bacteria to grow on its surface. Also always marinate meat in the refrigerator and when you have finished cooking make sure you get rid of any leftover marinade.

Tip 6 – Make sure that your barbecue grill has been preheated before you start cooking on it. If you are using a gas model then allow around 10 to 15 minutes for it to get up to the correct temperature. If however you are using a charcoal model then allow this around 30 minutes to reach the temperature required for cooking.

Plus make sure that you adjust the temperature to suit the kind of food you will be cooking on yours. For example if you are going to be cooking steaks or other cuts of meat on yours make sure that you keep the temperature as high as possible. Whilst lower the heat when cooking items such as vegetables or fish.

Tip 7 – It is important that you cook similar sized pieces of food together at the same time. This will then help to ensure that everything cooks evenly. Plus make sure that you turn food often to further ensure that each piece is cooked through evenly. If you notice that food is starting to burn then move the grate up away from the heat source or by reducing the heat. To reduce the heat being produced by charcoal either damp them down by spraying with some water, remember to move food out of the way first, or by closing the air vents partially.

Tip 8 – Never cook anything from frozen on a barbecue grill. The problem is that it can cause permanent damage to the surface of the grate.

Tip 9 – You should trim any excess fat from the meat you are cooking, as well as cut slits into the remaining fat at two inch intervals. Not only will this prevent flare ups from occurring but also will help to prevent the meat from curling up. Furthermore applying some salt after cooking will then help to prevent the meat from drying out.

Tip 10 – When cooking chicken on a barbecue grill you need to be very careful. To test to make sure that it is cooked through you can either place a meat thermometer into it? Ideally when you stick a thermometer into chicken the internal temperature should be between 170 and 175 degrees Fahrenheit to ensure that it being cooked inside correctly. However the quickest and simplest way of seeing whether the meat is cooked or not is to make an incision (cut) into the thickest part of the chicken. If you notice it is still pink inside then place it back on to the barbecue until when you look inside the cut again you notice it is white all the way through.

Tip 11 – Make sure that you keep all food well covered both before and after it has been cooked. If you don't then flies may well land on it and leave behind bacteria that could make you and others ill.

Tip 12 – Finally never leave food that has been cooked hanging around at room temperature. If you do there is an opportunity for bacteria to grow on it. After cooking keep the food close to the heat source or once cooled down place it in the refrigerator.

If you follow the rules provided above then of course you will find that not only food tastes a great deal better, but also you are reducing the risk of causing harm to those who attend your barbecue. Plus of course you will all have a much more enjoyable time.

Chapter 5 - Cooking On A Barbecue

As you know when it comes to cooking on a barbecue you need to be very careful. There are certain things to remember if you don't then you are putting the health of those who come to your barbecue at risk. Here are some words of advice you should heed when it comes to cooking on a barbecue.

1. It is important before you begin cooking that you check that the right temperature has been reached. If it isn't at the right temperature you could end up over or under cooking the food. Although some barbecues are now fitted with a thermometer to tell you what the temperature is inside the less expensive models don't come with such features.
   The best way for you to check the temperature is to put your hand above the grate palm side down. If you are only able to hold your hand over the heat for 2 seconds then this tells you the temperature is hot. However if you are able to hold your hand over the barbecue for between 3 and 4 seconds you barbecue is producing medium to hot heat. Whilst if you can hold your hand over the barbecue for 4 to 5 seconds then heat has reached a medium temperature.
2. When it comes to cooking on a barbecue you need to be patient, both when it is heating up and when you need it to cool down. If you don't allow sufficient time for the barbecue to

heat up or cool down you won't be able to cook the food properly.

3. If flare-ups occur when cooking then move the food away from the area concerned for a few minutes and sprinkle some water lightly over the flames. It is a good idea to have a spray bottle close at hand filled with water than you can use to help dampen down flare-ups as soon as they occur.

4. When it comes to cooking meat you should allow dark meat such as steak to cook on your barbecue for around 30 minutes. Whereas white meat such as poultry should be cooked for around 15 minutes. During this time make sure that you turn the meat over at least once every five minutes or so.

5. If you are going to be using any marinade as a sauce then make sure that you cook it before you use it. This will then help to prevent any kind of cross contamination occurring. Ideally cook the marinade until it reaches a temperature of 140 degrees Fahrenheit as this will help to ensure that any microbes or bacteria in it taken from the raw food are killed off.

Samantha Michaels

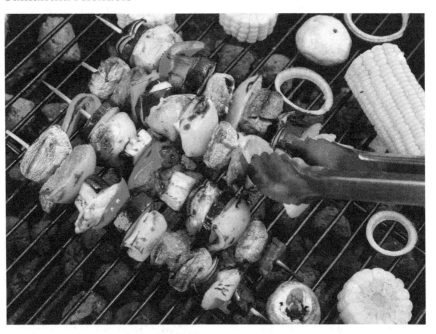

Chapter 6 - Quick & Simple Barbecue Recipes To Try

If you aren't sure what to cook on your barbecue below are some very quick and simple recipes you may want to consider trying.

Recipe 1	Barbecued Baby Back Ribs
Recipe 2	Gilled Steak
Recipe 3	Grilled Chicken Breast
Recipe 4	Grilled Chicken Wings
Recipe 5	Grilled Lamb Chops
Recipe 6	Grilled Pork Chops
Recipe 7	Grilled Salmon
Recipe 8	Grilled Shrimp
Recipe 9	Halloumi Kebabs
Recipe 10	Chocolate Baked Bananas

Recipe 1 – Barbecued Baby Back Ribs

Ingredients

- Baby Back Ribs
- 2 Tablespoons Unsalted Meat Tenderizer
- 2 Tablespoons Cayenne Pepper
- 1 Tablespoon Seasoning Salt
- 2 Tablespoons Paprika
- 1 ½ Tablespoons Onion Powder
- 1 ½ Tablespoons Garlic Powder
- 1 Tablespoon Black Pepper

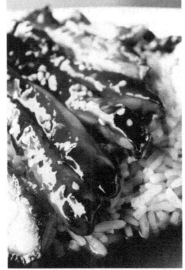

Step 1 – Into a small bowl you should mix equal amounts of the meat tenderizer, cayenne pepper, salt, paprika, garlic and onion powder and black pepper. It is important to make sure that all these ingredients are mixed thoroughly together and then place them into an empty shaker. Before using make sure that you shake the ingredients well and any seasoning left over should be stored somewhere cool and dry.

Step 2 – Make sure that you shake the seasoning over the ribs covering them all evenly. Once this has done then place them over night in the fridge to allow the flavors of the seasoning to infuse into the meat. Remember to cover the meat over when stored in the refrigerator and place on the bottom shelf.

Step 3 – Before you cook your ribs you should take them out of the fridge a short while before so that they can come to room temperature. In fact whilst they are coming up to room temperature this is when you should be turning the barbecue on.

Step 4 – When starting up your barbecue make sure that the coals are prepared for direct heat cooking. Ideally the grate should be around 3 inches above the heat source.

Step 5 – As soon as the barbecue is hot enough now you can put the baby back ribs onto cook. You need to place them on the grate bone side down first. It is important that once your ribs do start to cook that you actually turn them often and to help prevent them from drying out make sure that you baste them regular. Your baste mixture should be made up of some of the seasoning in which the ribs were marinated the night before to which you add some water and vinegar.

Step 6 – Once the ribs are cooked you can either coat them in your favorite barbecue sauce for a few minutes or you can eat them as they are.

Recipe 2 - Grilled Steak

Ingredients

- Steak (Rib Eye, Sirloin Or Fillet would be best)
- ½ Cup Olive Oil
- 1 Tablespoon Salt
- 1 ½ Tablespoon Pepper

To cook the perfect steak each time on your barbecue grill to ensure it remains juicy and full of flavor you need to carry out the following steps.

Step 1 – Once the barbecue has reached the desired temperature now need to brush both sides of the steak with some olive oil as this will help to prevent it from sticking to the grate. Also by brushing the steak rather than the grate you are preventing the oil from burning, which could not only cause a lot of smoke to be produced but also flare-ups.

Step 2 – Just before you actually put the stakes on the barbecue to cook season them with some salt and pepper. Only season the meat one side at the time before cooking as this will then help to seal in more of the flavor. Also don't apply too much salt as this can help to draw out too many of the meats juices and will make it tough to eat. Season the second side of the meat with salt and pepper just before you are going to cook it.

Step 3 – Cook the steak on the barbecue using a set of long handled tongs to help turn it over. Also only ever turn the steak over once if you turn it more than this more of the juices will escape and again will make the meat much tougher to eat.

Step 4 – Once the meat has finished cooking depending on how people like it and how thick it is you need to place it on a clean plate and cover with foil. Now set aside for 5 minutes to rest as this will allow for more of the juices to be pushed to the center of the meat and will also help it to relax, in turn this will make it taste more succulent and tender.

If you have never cooked steak on a barbecue before you make find these timing guidelines of some use. For steak that is 1.5 cm thick you should cook the meat for the following amounts of time.

1. Rare Steak – Cook for 1 to 1 ½ minutes on each side
2. Medium Steak – Cook for 2 to 3 minutes on each side
3. Well Done Steak – Cook for 3 to 4 minutes on each side

For steak that is 2 to 3 cm thick you should cook the meat for the following amount of time.

1. Rare Steak – 2 to 3 minutes on each side
2. Medium Steak – 4 to 5 minutes on each side
3. Well Done Steak – 5 to 6 minutes on each side

Recipe 3 – Grilled Chicken Breast

Ingredients

- 3 or 4 Chicken Breasts (Free range or organic are best)
- ½ Cup Olive Oil
- ¼ Cup Lemon Juice
- 1 ½ Tablespoons Freshly Ground Black Pepper
- 1 Tablespoon Salt
- 1 Clove Of Garlic Minced
- ¼ Cup Finely Chopped Onion
- ¼ Teaspoon Thyme (Fresh is best, but dried will do)
- 1/8 Teaspoon Cumin

To create this very simple grilled chicken breast you need to carry out the following steps.

Step 1 – Into a bowl place all the ingredients mentioned above to make the marinade. Then once they have all been combined well together place them into a strong plastic bag. Choose a bag that will allow you to seal up the top.

Step 2 – Once the marinade is ready you now add the chicken breasts to them in the back and seal the bag up. Now place in the refrigerator for the next 6 to 8 hours to left the chicken become infused with the marinade. It is important that every two hours you actually turn the bag over so that the marinade is able to cover all parts of the chicken breast.

Step 3 – After the allotted time (6 to 8 hours) your chicken breasts are ready to cook. If you are using a charcoal barbecue grill make sure that coals are at the right temperature they should be glowing red. When the coals are hot enough you can now start cooking the chicken breasts on the grill. It is important that the barbecue grill grate is set at least 6 inches above the coals. This will ensure that the exterior of the breasts doesn't get burnt or that the chicken breasts won't dry out.

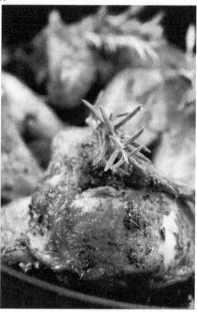

Step 4 – To make sure that the chicken is cooked through properly either insert the probe of a meat thermometer into the breasts. If the interior of the meat has reached a temperature of 165 degrees Fahrenheit it should be cooked through. The other simple way to check if the meat is cooked through if you don't have a meat thermometer is to insert a skewer and when withdrawn do the juices that run out of the meat run clear.

Step 5 – Once the chicken is cooked you should remove it from the barbecue grill and then allow it to cool for a few seconds. Once cooled you can then start eating it either on its own or in a bun with your favorite condiment and a salad.

Recipe 4 – Grilled Chicken Wings

Ingredients

- 12 Chicken Wings
- ½ Cup Soy Sauce
- ¼ Cup Honey
- ¼ Cup Tomato Sauce
- ¼ Cup White Wine Vinegar
- 1 Glove of Garlic Minced
- 1 Teaspoon Ground Ginger
- Pinch Of Chilli Powder

This like all the other recipes in this book is very easy to make and will provide you with some very delicious tasting food for your next barbecue. To make this particular recipe the steps you need to carry out are as follows:

Step 1 – Rinse the chicken wings thoroughly by placing them under cold running water. Once they have been thoroughly rinsed you need to pat them dry using some paper towel and set them aside for use in a little while. Remember to keep them covered up to prevent any germs or bacteria from forming on them.

Step 2 – Into a bowl (non metallic preferably) that is large enough to hold all the chicken wings in a single layer mix together the ingredients mentioned above to create the marinade. Once it has been made you must put aside at least a ¼ cup of the marinade, as you will be using this for basting the chicken wings when they are cooking on the barbecue.

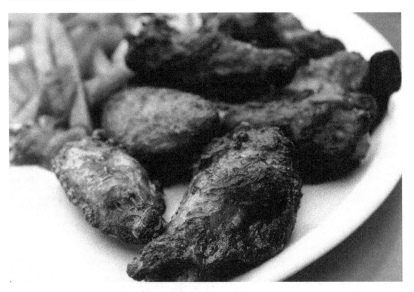

Step 3 – After removing ¼ cup of the marinade from the bowl you can add the chicken wings to the mixture. Make sure that you turn the wings thoroughly through the mixture to ensure that every part of them is coated with the marinade. When this is done cover the top of the bowl with cling film or aluminum foil before placing in the refrigerator and leaving them to become infused with the marinade overnight.

Step 4 – When you are ready to grill yours on the barbecue then you can remove them from the marinade. It is important that you place the grate for the barbecue grill at least six inches above the heat source and that the heat is at a medium temperature. Be aware that to ensure that the chicken wings are cooked properly will take around 35 to 40 minutes and you will have to spend time turning them over regularly to prevent them from becoming burnt or drying out.

Recipe 5 – Grilled Lamb Chop

Ingredients

- Lamb Chops That Are Around An Inch Thick
- ½ Teaspoon Fresh Rosemary For Each Chop (However if you cannot get hold of fresh rosemary dried will do)
- ½ Tablespoon Olive Oil For Each Chop
- Pinch of Salt and Pepper For Each Chop

Although lamb is quite expensive it tastes absolutely wonderful when grilled on a barbecue. To make this recipe you need to carry out the following steps.

Step 1 – First of you need to trim off some if not all the fat on the chop. By doing this you are helping to reduce the risk of flare ups occurring once you start cooking the chops on your barbecue grill. Also removing it won't actually make the chops taste any different, as it doesn't add any flavor to it when cooking. The fat that does add flavor is that which you will see throughout the chop.

Step 2 – After trimming of the excess fat you need to rinse the chops under running cold water and then pat dry using paper towels. Once this is done you now need to brush both sides of the chop with the olive oil before you then sprinkle on to them the rosemary, salt and pepper. After doing this place on a clean plate and cover with aluminum foil before placing in the refrigerator for ½ hour.

Step 3 – Whilst you are waiting for the barbecue to heat up to the correct temperature remove the chops from the refrigerator, leaving them covered up so that they can come up to room temperature. If you are going to be using a gas barbecue to cook your lamb chops on leave the lid closed for about 10 to 15 minutes before you are going to start cooking. This will help the grate on which the lamb chops to become a lot hotter and as result will leave those wonderful grill marks on the surface of the meat. Plus it will also add to the radiant heat, which will help to make sure that the chops will be cooked more evenly.

Step 4 – As soon as the barbecue grill is ready you should remove the grate so that you can then very carefully oil it with some vegetable oil that is on a paper towel. Now place the grate back in position.

Step 5 – Now place the chops on the grate and grill them over a high heat with the lid open. Should any flare-ups occur whilst cooking then simply move the chops over to an area of the grate where the heat isn't as great until the flames have died down. After around 4 minutes you now need to turn the chops over and then cook them on the other side for around 4 minutes. Of course you may need to cook them for longer or shorter on each side dependent on the thickness of the chops, what the exterior temperature is like and what the temperature within the barbecue is.

Step 6 – When the chops are cooked as required you should let them rest for a short while (around 5 minutes) before serving. Remember to keep them covered whilst they are resting.

Recipe 6 – Grilled Pork Chop

Ingredients

- 4 Boneless Pork Loin Chops
- ¼ Cup Olive Oil
- 2 ½ Tablespoons Soy Sauce
- 1 Teaspoon Steak Seasoning

Although this is a very quick and simple recipe to use when you want to grill pork chops on a barbecue you will find that they taste wonderful. To make this recipe you need to carry out the following steps.

Step 1 – In a small bowl mix together the olive oil, soy sauce and steak seasoning. Once these ingredients have been mixed together thoroughly you now need to pour them into a strong plastic bag that can be sealed. This is the marinade for coating the pork chops and which makes them taste so wonderful.

Step 2 – Once you have poured the marinade into the bag you are now ready to add the pork. But before you do rinse them thoroughly under cold running water and then pat dry using some paper towels. After adding the chops to the marinade mixture in the bag you now place it sealed in to a baking dish ensuring that each chop is laid flat so that they all get an equal amount of the marinade coating them. If you want to ensure that the marinade infuses well into the meat then flip the bag over once half way through the marinating time.

Step 3 – After laying them in the bag in the baking dish you now need to put the chops into the refrigerator and let them remain in the marinade for between 3 to 8 hours.

Step 4 – After the allotted time is up you should remove the chops from the refrigerator still in the bag and let them come up to room temperature. Whilst this is happening you can actually get the barbecue on to ensure that it is then at the right temperature for cooking the chops.

Step 5 – You need to ensure that when cooking the chops on the barbecue it is only on a medium heat and each chop should be grilled for 6 to 8 minutes on each side. How long they are cooked for on each side of course depends on how thick the chops are. If you can make an incision in one of the chops to check to see if the center is no longer pink. If it is then keep on the barbecue for a little longer.

Step 6 – Once the chops have been cooked through thoroughly remove from the grate and place them on a clean plate and cover with aluminum foil. Then allow them to rest for between 5 to 7 minutes before serving to your guests.

Recipe 7 – Grilled Salmon

Ingredients
4 x 1 to 1 ¼ Inch Thick Fresh Or Frozen Salmon
Fillets
¼ Cup Cooking Oil (Olive Would Be Best)
¼ Cup Orange Juice
¼ Cup Dry White Wine
3 Tablespoons Of Freshly Snipped Parsley
2 Cloves Garlic Minced
¼ Teaspoon Salt
Dash Of Pepper

To make this particular recipe that will allow you to serve your guests with beautiful tasting salmon at your next barbecue you need to carry out the following.

Step 1 – If you are using frozen salmon fillets then make sure that they are defrosted completely. However if you want your salmon to taste really wonderful you should use fresh salmon whenever possible.

Step 2 – Place the salmon fillets in a shallow dish. One that is large enough to accommodate all the fillets so that there is space between them. Cover and put to one side whilst you make the marinade for them.

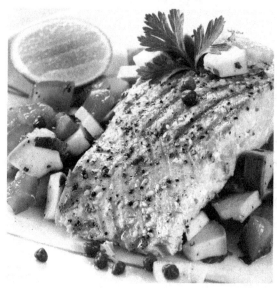

Step 3 – To make the marinade you need a small bowl into which you then pour the oil, orange juice, dry white wine, parsley, garlic, salt and pepper. Mix together with a whisk before then pouring over the salmon. Then turn each fillet of salmon over to ensure that the fillets have been thoroughly coated in the marinade.

Step 4 – Cover the salmon fillets in the dish once more before then placing into the refrigerator for between 6 to 24 hours. Make sure that you actually turn over the fillets several times whilst they remain in the refrigerator. This will then help more of the marinade to be absorbed by them.

Step 5 – When it comes time to cook the fillets you should drain them first and pat them with paper towels to remove any excess moisture. Any marinade that is left over place to one side as you can then use this to baste the fillets when they are cooking.

Step 6 – To cook them on the barbecue you should place them on a grate over a medium heat and cook them on each side for between 6 to 8 minutes. If cooked properly when you test them with a fork the salmon meat should flake easily. When cooking make sure that you brush the fillets regularly with the marinade left over.

Recipe 8 – Grilled Shrimp

Ingredients

- 2 lbs of Fresh Tiger or Jumper Shrimp (before you begin cooking you need to peel and devein them)
- ½ Cup Fresh Lemon Juice (This will come from about 3 medium size lemons)
- ½ Cup Olive Oil
- ¼ Cup Fresh Parsley
- ¼ Cup Green Onions
- 3 Gloves Garlic Minced
- 3 Tablespoons Soy Sauce
- 2 Tablespoons Sesame Oil

Although the actual time it takes to prepare and cook the shrimps isn't very long. If you want yours to be infused with as much of the marinade flavor as possible you need to leave the shrimp in it for as long as possible. To create this wonderful tasting food for your barbecue you need to carry out the following.

Step 1 – Into a bowl pour the fresh lemon juice, olive oil, parsley, garlic, onions, and soy sauce and sesame oil. Once you have put all these ingredients into the bowl make sure that they are thoroughly combined by whisking them together vigorously.

Step 2 – Once the marinade mixture is ready you can now add the shrimps to them. It is best to use your hands to make sure that each shrimp you put into the bowl is fully coated in the marinade. Now place the bowl, which you have covered into the refrigerator and leave the marinade to soak into the shrimps for around 3 to 4 hours before you cook them. Whilst in the refrigerator stir the shrimps at least twice.

Step 3 – When it is near time to start cooking the shrimps on the barbecue then prepare it for direct cooking. The grate on which you are cooking the shrimps should be well oiled and positioned between 4 and 6 inches above the heat source. When the desired temperature has been reached you are now ready to place the shrimps onto the grate. Don't forget to take the shrimps out of the refrigerator at least 30 minutes before you intend to cook them.

Step 4 – When it comes to cooking the shrimps you need to remove them from the marinade and place on to the grate. Any marinade left in the bowl after removing all the shrimps can be used to baste them whilst they are cooking.

Step 5 – Each shrimp needs to be cooked on both sides for around 3 to 4 minutes. If you want to avoid them getting burnt it won't hurt to actually turn them after about a minute. Also it will also help to add more flavor to them if you baste them regularly in the marinade that remains in the bowl. You will know when the shrimps are done because they will have turned pink.

A great way of checking to see if the shrimps or done is to actually taste one. If you have cooked them for too long they will be very tough to eat and won't actually taste of anything.

Recipe 9 – Halloumi Kebabs

Ingredients
250g (8 ounces) Low Fat Halloumi Cheese that is cut into 16 chunks
2 Medium Size Courgettes
1 Large Red Onion
16 Cherry Tomatoes
1 Tablespoon Olive Oil
2 Tablespoon Lemon Juice
2 Tablespoon Fresh Thyme Leaves (If you can get hold of it use lemon thyme)
1 Teaspoon Dijon Mustard

This is the perfect recipe to use if you have any guests coming to your barbecue who happen to be vegetarians. Of course make sure that you cook these well away from any meat or fish you are cooking on the barbecue. It may be a good idea to actually cook these first and then place them in a warm oven whilst other items are cooking on the barbecue.

To make this particular food for your next barbecue you need to carry out the following steps.

Step 1 – Halve each of the courgettes lengthways before then cutting into thick slices. Cut the onion into wedges and then separate them up.

NOTE: If you are going to be using wooden skewers for making these kebabs then soak them in some water for around an hour as this will prevent them from burning.

Step 2 – On to each skewer (8 will be needed) you thread 2 chunks of Halloumi some cherry tomatoes, courgettes and onion.

Step 3 – After you have placed the above ingredients on to each of the skewers you now need to cover them and place them into the refrigerator until you are ready to cook them. You should only ever make these kebabs a few hours before the barbecue commences.

Step 4 – Once you have made the kebabs you are now ready to make the sauce which you will then baste them with whilst they are cooking. To make the sauce mix together the olive oil, lemon juice, thyme and mustard, along with any seasoning. Again like the kebabs you can actually prepare the sauce well before the barbecue commences.

Step 5 – To cook the kebabs you must make sure that you have the barbecue heated up properly before placing the kebabs on the grate. Remember to oil the grate well before cooking commences. Not only will this prevent the cheese from sticking to it but also help to create that lovely pattern on the surface of the food cooking.

Step 6 – Once you have placed the kebabs on the grate you need to brush on some of the basting sauce. Make sure that you stir it well to ensure that all the ingredients have been fully combined together and will provide the same flavor to all the kebabs.

Step 7 – Now cook each kebab for around 4 to 5 minutes making sure that you turn them over frequently and of course brushing them with the basting sauce each time you turn them. You will know when the kebabs are ready because the cheese will have turned a lovely golden brown color and the vegetables when touched will feel tender.

Step 8 – Once removed from the heat serve immediately with a crisp green salad and some warm pitta bread.

Recipe 10 – Chocolate Baked Bananas

Ingredients
4 Ripe Bananas
2 x 32g (1 ounce) Bag Chocolate Buttons

This is a wonderful dessert to serve at the end of your barbecue and is the easiest of all the recipes in this book to make.

To make this wonderful dessert you need to carry out the following.

Step 1 – Make a slit into the banana through the skin along one side. It is important that you don't cut all the way through.

Step 2 – After making the slit into the banana into this you now insert some of the chocolate buttons. Make sure that you insert them along the complete length of the cut made.

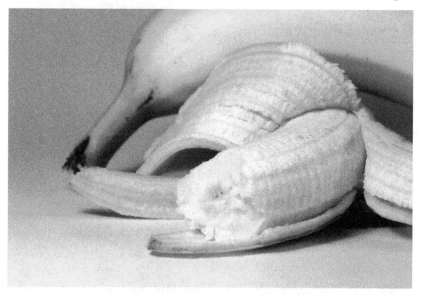

Step 3 – Place each of the bananas on a sheet of aluminum foil and now fold the edges over, crimping them together to ensure that the banana and chocolate buttons inside are completely sealed in.

Step 4 – Once you have covered the bananas in the tin foil place them in the embers of the barbecue and leave them for around 15 minutes.

Step 5 – As soon as the time has passed remove from the embers and undo the tin foil. The skin of the banana should have turned black by now.

Step 6 – To serve them remove from the aluminum foil onto a plate or into a dish and add a scoop of vanilla ice cream. Then eat.

MORE 70 BEST EVER RECIPES EBOOKS REVEALED AT MY AUTHOR PAGE:

CLICK HERE TO ACCESS THEM NOW

CPSIA information can be obtained
at www.ICGtesting.com
Printed in the USA
LVHW081053030123
736342LV00014B/419